D0984513

DARWINISM

TODAY

SHAPING LIFE

GENES, EMBRYOS AND EVOLUTION

John Maynard Smith

Weidenfeld & Nicolson
LONDON

First published in Great Britain in 1998 by
Weidenfeld & Nicolson
The Orion Publishing Group Ltd
Orion House
5 Upper Saint Martin's Lane
London, WC2H 9EA

A CIP catalogue record for this book is available
from the British Library.

ISBN 0 297 84138 6

Typeset by SetSystems Ltd, Saffron Walden, Essex

Set in 11/14.5 Bembo

Printed in Great Britain by Clays Ltd, St Ives plc

CONTENTS

The Series Editors thank
Colin Tudge, Peter Holland, Damon de Laszlo
and Peter Tallack for their help.

FOREWORD

Darwinism Today is a series of short books by leading figures in the field of evolutionary theory. Each title is an authoritative pocket introduction to the Darwinian ideas that are setting today's intellectual agenda.

The series developed out of the Darwin@LSE programme at the London School of Economics. The Darwin Seminars provide a platform for distinguished evolutionists to present the latest Darwinian thinking and to explore its application to humans. The programme is having an enormous impact, both in helping to popularize evolutionary theory, and in fostering cross-disciplinary approaches to shared problems.

With the publication of **Darwinism Today** we hope that the best of the new Darwinian ideas will reach an even wider audience.

Helena Cronin and Oliver Curry
Series Editors

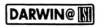

SHAPING LIFE

GENES, EMBRYOS AND EVOLUTION

CHAPTER I

....

Development:
The Recent Revolution

During the past ten years, there has been a revolution in our understanding of development, the process whereby an egg turns into an adult organism. As yet, this revolution has been little appreciated outside biology, perhaps because the research has been so exciting that the people engaged have had little time to explain what is happening to a wider audience. This is a pity, because the change from a simple undifferentiated egg into a complex adult is fascinating, and was, until recently, mysterious. When, some fifteen years ago, I wrote a book called *The Problems of Biology*, I identified this process as one of the two major problem areas of biology, along with how the brain works.[1]

If I were to rewrite that book today, I would not treat development as a major problem area, but rather as one in which there is dramatic progress towards a solution. This progress is being made by applying the ideas and techniques of genetics to the processes of development. The philosophy behind this approach is that the genes carry, in digital form, the instructions for making an organism. It is a philosophy that traces back to the Austrian biologist Gregor Johann Mendel (1822–84), and the idea that there are, within the egg, factors that influence the development of particular parts or organs. My main aim in this book is to give a brief account of the revolution that is happening. But I want also to refer to another tradition, which sees development in more holistic terms. The roots of this tradition trace back to the *Naturphilosophie* of Johann Wolfgang von Goethe (1749–1832). Today, it is represented by the notion of 'self-organization', and is supported by reference to the complex patterns that can emerge in dynamical systems, without the need for specific instructions regulating the development of particular parts. Developmental geneticists, confident in the successes that their methods are achieving, tend to ignore this alternative tradition. They may be right. But there are observations suggesting that we should pay attention to dynamical processes as well as to genetic control; some of these observations are described below. Ultimately, I think that some dialogue will be needed. If this book contributes to encouraging such dialogue, I shall be delighted.

I am not myself an embryologist, but an evolutionary biologist. There is a parallel, long appreciated, between the *developmental* changes that convert an egg into an adult, and the *evolutionary* changes that, on an enormously longer time scale, have converted simple single-celled ancestors into the existing array of multicellular animals and plants. In both cases, a single cell is converted into an organism with many cells, of many different kinds, arranged in a complex three-dimensional structure. But, despite the similarity, the mechanisms are entirely different: development is not driven by natural selection. All the same, the two processes are intimately connected. Development depends on genetic information that has been accumulated over millions of years of evolution, and the evolution of adult forms has depended on developmental changes in successive generations.

Ever since I was a student of zoology, almost fifty years ago, people have been saying that evolutionary biology would be transformed once we had an understanding of embryology. I have even said so myself. Evolutionary theory is largely concerned with changes in the frequencies of genes in populations, brought about by mutation, natural selection and other processes. What we observe in evolution are changes in the forms of animals and plants. To link theory and observation, we need to know how changes in genes cause changes in morphology, and that requires an understanding of development. Until recently, however, little light has been shed on evolution by students of development. There has been much talk of the way in which development constrains the kinds of evolutionary novelty that can arise in particular lineages. This is no doubt true; but merely using the phrase 'developmental constraint' does not help much if one cannot specify what the constraints are or why they exist. For example, it is a curious fact that monocotyledonous plants (eg. lilies or daffodils) almost always have flower parts (petals, sepals) in rings of three, whereas dicots (eg. buttercups or roses) typically have rings of four, five or more. This can hardly be explained by natural selection, because the two groups of flowering plants have access to identical pollinating insects. Presumably the difference has to do with a difference in the mechanisms of flower development. But this is not very illuminating if we do not know what that difference is.

I believe that things are now changing, in the main because of progress in developmental genetics. In classical genetics, the existence of a gene is deduced from the analysis of families in which mutant forms of the gene are present, producing individuals with changed characteristics. In developmental genetics, an attempt is made to discover how mutant genes cause their effects, and to deduce what the unmutated gene does in normal development. New molecular techniques enable us to identify genes that are active early in development, to determine their DNA sequence, to discover where and when they are active, and to study the effects of inactivating such genes, or causing them to be activated in unusual positions in the embryo, or even of transferring them to members of other phyla. New information is being discovered at a bewildering rate. As yet, it is difficult to see the wood for the trees. Just what is the significance of this revolution in developmental genetics for evolution?

A second strand that may perhaps have some relevance to development has a completely different origin. Increases in computer power have made it relatively easy to study the behaviour of complex systems. It has become apparent that 'dynamic systems' governed by rather simple rules can give rise to very complex results, and in particular to complex spatial patterns (the behaviour of the weather and waves on the surface of water are familiar examples). The idea of drawing parallels between biological forms and the forms generated by physical systems is of course not new − it was, for example, the inspiration of the Scottish biologist D'Arcy Thompson (1860−1948) in his book *On Growth and Form* (1917) − but recent simulations of dynamical systems have given it a new lease of life.

At present, workers in these two fields − developmental genetics and complex systems − communicate rather rarely. Developmental geneticists see little need to invoke complex dynamics when they are getting on quite nicely without them. With a few honourable exceptions, students of complex systems appear to think that development can best be studied by ignoring the facts of biology, and forgetting about the only serious theoretical idea we have – the idea of natural selection that originates with Charles Darwin (1809–82). Yet I think it possible that a proper understanding of development will need *both* approaches. I have no doubt at all that recent genetic studies have provided an essential insight into development. They also provide the necessary link between development and evolution: natural selection explains how information is incorporated in the genome, and development shows what use is made of it during the development of each individual. But there are some observations that suggest that a dynamic systems approach will also be needed. In this book, I want to attempt two things: first, to explain the central ideas to a wider public in non-technical language, and second, perhaps to persuade a few people working in one school or the other to consider communicating across the divide.

CHAPTER 2

....

The Conservation of Signals

The essence of the revolution in developmental genetics is shown by the results of a remarkable experiment.[2] In the mouse, there is a gene called 'small-eye'. If this gene mutates, it causes the development of a mouse without eyes. What this means, of course, is that the gene, in its normal unmutated form, plays a necessary role in the development of the eye. If the gene mutates it no longer does its job and no eye develops. If the normal form of this gene is transferred to the developing fruitfly, *Drosophila*, and is then activated, it causes the development of an eye wherever it is activated – not, of course, a mouse eye, but a compound *Drosophila* eye, with the characteristic facets. The natural interpretation is that the gene that induces the development of an eye at a particular place in the mouse is sufficiently similar to the gene that does the same job in *Drosophila* that the one can replace the other. This interpretation is confirmed by the fact that the two genes are very similar in the sequence of their nucleotides, and hence in the nature of the proteins that they specify. This in turn makes it very likely that the common ancestor of mouse and fly already possessed a light-sensitive organ – perhaps no more than a few light-sensitive cells – and that the development of this organ at a particular place was induced by a gene ancestral to those now present in mouse and fly. If so, the gene, which can be thought of as a signal saying 'make an eye here', has been conserved in sequence, despite the fact that the kind of eye made in response to the signal is wholly different in mouse and fly. The fact that very different eye structures, the compound eye of a fly and the camera-like eye of vertebrates, can be specified by very similar signals should not surprise us – after all, one can use a similar switch for turning on a television set or a light bulb. What is curious is the conservation of the signal for at least six hundred million years.

Even if we accept the common ancestry of the control genes for eye development in insects and vertebrates, it is important to remember that there is little in common between the structure of their eyes, and that eyes evolved independently in the two groups and, indeed, in many other animals. The question, then, is what the regulatory genes were doing before they controlled the location of eye development. They may have been controlling the appearance of simple light-sensitive cells, or even of some other type of sensory cell. This is an example of a more general problem. Biologists say that two structures are 'homologous' if they are derived by a series of evolutionary transformations from the same structure in a common ancestor. In this sense, human arms and bird wings are homologous, but insect and vertebrate eyes are usually thought not to be. Two genes are said to be homologous if they are derived by replication from the same gene in a common ancestor: homology of genes is deduced from similarity of base sequence. Can we deduce that two structures are homologous if they are induced by homologous genes? The example of eyes suggests that we cannot. But surely a common genetic control must count as evidence in favour of homology? This is one of the many unanswered questions raised by recent work in developmental genetics.

In mice there is a series of genes, the Hox genes, linearly arranged along the chromosome, that are activated in sequence early in development from the anterior to the posterior region of the embryo. These genes can also be thought of as switches, activating other genes, and so inducing appropriate structures to develop. It is a curious feature, not well understood, that the sequence of these genes along the chromosome corresponds to their sequence of activity along the body axis from front to back, so that the first gene on the chromosome is active in the most anterior region of the embryo, and so on along the chromosome. In *Drosophila* there is a similar set of Hox genes, also arranged linearly; in this case, in two groups, on two separate chromosomes. They are active early in the developing embryo, with sites of activity varying from the front to the rear of the embryo, in the same sequence as the genes are arranged along the chromosome. By their activity they induce the development of the appropriate structures antero-posteriorly – for example, antennae, wings, genitalia. Each Hox gene codes for a 'homeodomain'; this is a region of some sixty amino acids at the start of the protein, which acts to regulate other genes. An astonishing fact emerged when the precise sequences of these homeobox regions were determined. It turns out that the most anteriorly-acting of the mouse genes is more similar to the most anteriorly-acting of the fly genes than it is to any of the genes in the mouse series; and so on along the sequence. It has since been discovered that a similar series of homeobox genes exists in all the main bilaterally symmetrical animal phyla, including molluscs (eg. snails, octopus) and annelid worms (eg. earthworms, leeches). Again, we are forced to the conclusion that a signalling system has been conserved, although the structures that it induces are quite different. Indeed, it has been suggested that this system is the common, primitive feature shared by all animals: the kingdom Animalia can be defined as including all organisms that possess this signalling system.[3]

I cannot resist a digression at this point to mention the 'Great Debate' in 1830 at the French Academy between the biologist Geoffroy St Hilaire (1772–1844) and the comparative anatomist Georges Cuvier (1769–1832).[4] Geoffroy was the protagonist for 'philosophical anatomy', confronted by the more empirically motivated Cuvier. Geoffroy argued for the unity of the animal kingdom and the possibility of drawing parallels among the morphologies of all animals. For reasons that today we find rather difficult to grasp, Geoffroy saw this morphological unity of all animals as having great philosophical significance. In contrast, Cuvier argued for the existence of four 'embranchements' – vertebrates, arthropods, molluscs and echinoderms – within which parallels could be drawn but between which they were impossible. At the time, the general feeling was that Cuvier's superior empirical knowledge had won him the debate. Today we might be tempted to reverse that judgement. In one respect, we would certainly incline to do so. Geoffroy found it hard to draw parallels between the arthropods and vertebrates, because the arthropods have a ventral nerve cord, and the vertebrates a dorsal one. He solved the problem by suggesting that the vertebrates were arthropods upside down. I remember this being related to me when I was a student as an illustration of how stupid past scientists (particularly, it was hinted, if they were French) could be. Recently, the discovery of genes determining the dorso-ventral axis in vertebrates and insects has suggested that Geoffroy may have been right after all.[5] There is a gene, *sog*, in *Drosophila* that determines ventral development: in the toad, *Xenopus*, a similar gene, *chordin*, determines dorsal development. It has been shown that these two genes are functionally equivalent by injecting mRNA transcript (see Chapter 4) of *sog* into a toad, where it induced dorsal development, and injecting mRNA from the gene *chordin* into *Drosophila*, where it induced ventral development. In other words, the same signal that induces ventral development in an insect induces dorsal development in a vertebrate. Does this prove that the ancestral vertebrates were relatives of the ancestors of the insects which adopted the habit of swimming upside down? The suggestion is not absurd: there are insects today (the back-swimming water boatmen) that live upside down, relative to other insects. In the light of these recent genetic findings, I cannot help imagining Geoffroy, wherever he may now be, shaking his finger at Cuvier and saying, 'I told you so.' But if Geoffroy was right, it was not in the way he thought. If anything has been conserved, it is not morphology but a signalling system: not form but information.

For an evolutionary biologist, the puzzling feature of these findings concerning the Hox genes and the *eyeless* gene – and many other examples could have been given – is the extraordinary conservatism of the genes that act as signals inducing structures to develop at particular places, despite profound changes in the structures induced. Why conserve signals? One can understand why the form of an eye or a wing, or for that matter of an enzyme catalysing a particular reaction, should be conserved: to function properly, an eye or a wing must have a particular form. But a signal does not have to have a particular form. In human language, although speech is ancient, the actual words we use to denote particular things change rapidly. Indeed, we know that signalling genes can gain new functions as well as retaining old ones. Sometimes, in evolution, genes are duplicated. When this happens to genes coding for 'house-keeping' enzymes – that is, enzymes carrying out chemical reactions needed in all cells – the usual result is the degeneration and loss of one copy. But in the case of genes active in development, the new copy often acquires a new role: for example, in mammals the Hox genes have been duplicated, and the new copies are now active in limb development. So there is a real problem. Signals are conserved, although it should be easy for a signal to change its meaning, and although there is evidence that, after duplication, signalling genes can acquire additional meanings.

The obvious explanation of signal conservation is an evolutionary one. If evolution by natural selection is to lead to adaptive change (rather than merely conserve adaptations already present) it must be true that each step increases the chance of survival, if only by a little. It is not enough that the final result of many genetic mutations should be a new adaptive structure, if each mutation by itself is no use. Evolution has no foresight, and cannot incorporate the first changes unless they are adaptive, or at least not harmful. In the current jargon, evolution by natural selection is a hill-climbing process, and every step must be uphill. The same problem confronts those who design new machines by simulating evolution by natural selection on a computer. A necessary condition for hill-climbing is that mutational steps (or a significant proportion of them) should be small: large leaps are likely to be leaps into the abyss. Applied to signalling genes, this implies that, if you have a cascade of regulatory genes, with A switching on (or off) genes B, C and D, which then switch on E, F, G and H, and so on, the one gene you don't muck about with is gene A.

In other words, evolution by natural selection has ensured that signals acting early in development are conserved. It is important to be clear about what is being said here. It would not be true to say that signals are conserved *because* this ensures that organisms are 'evolvable': that is, so constructed that evolution is possible. This would imply that organisms have features that exist because they permit future evolution to occur: it would be another example of assuming evolutionary foresight. Instead, I am arguing that the only changes in signalling systems that happen in evolution are those that produce relatively small changes in morphology, and that these would not include changes in signals acting early in development.

Another, more familiar, type of conservation in evolution may have a similar explanation, although, as I will explain, there are difficulties. It has been recognized for some time that, during development, the members of a given phylum – for example, chordates (our own phylum) or echinoderms (starfish and sea urchins) – pass through a conserved 'phylotypic stage', a stage reminiscent of their ancient ancestors. For example, fish, mammals and birds all pass through a stage at which the embryo has a stiff rod along its back (the notochord), above which lies a hollow nerve cord, and either side of which are blocks of cells, the somites, which will develop into segmental muscles and skeletal elements (for example, vertebrae and ribs). The anterior part of the gut – the 'pharynx' – is perforated by a series of openings, which in fish will become the gill slits. In the early days of evolutionary theory, this close resemblance between the embryos of animals that would later grow into very different adults was interpreted in terms of 'recapitulation' – the idea that, during development, animals recapitulate their evolutionary history: they 'climb their own ancestral tree'. This idea has been abandoned for two reasons. First, there is no good reason why animals *should* recapitulate their evolutionary history. Second, and more important, it was realized that, early in development before the phylotypic stage, related animals may be more different from one another than they are later. This early variation is an adaptation to the process of development itself: for example, development is very different if the starting point is a large yolky egg like that of a bird or a shark than if the egg is small and lacking in yolk. Thus very different patterns of early cell division and migration may converge on a common phylotypic stage, and diverge again after it. We are left with the problem of why a common phylotypic stage has been conserved.[6]

A hint is given by the fact that early development is global to the whole embryo, and involves extensive cell movements. At the phylotypic stage, the main adult organs are already represented by blocks of undifferentiated cells, arranged in the appropriate relative positions. Later development of the different blocks is to a considerable degree independent, although signals do pass between them. Conservatism of the phylotypic stage again looks like a feature required if evolution is to proceed in small steps: it makes it easier for a change in a gene to alter one part without requiring changes in all other parts. For much the same reason, computer programmers tend to divide their programs into subroutines, any one of which can be modified without interfering with all the others. I think this is correct, but one must again be careful not to endow evolution with foresight, and argue that development is modular because it makes possible future evolution. I think, rather, that development is modular because that is the most efficient way of generating an organism: the reason for this will emerge later. However, the fact that it *is* modular makes continued evolution possible. It also helps to explain why the phylotypic stage is conserved.

Evolution has proceeded by modifying the later stages of development of individual modules, one at a time, while leaving the initial arrangement of those modules unaltered.

CHAPTER 3

....

Genetic Instructions

I must now return to the discussion of developmental genetics. The picture that is emerging is of a hierarchy of regulatory genes, active at specific times and at particular places, and acting to switch other genes on or off. The notion of 'gene switching' has been familiar since the work of the French biochemists François Jacob (1920–) and Jacques Monod (1910–76).[7] Like the discovery by James Watson and Francis Crick of the structure of DNA, this work is one of the foundation stones of molecular biology. Jacob and Monod were interested in the fact that a group of linked genes in the bacterium *Escherichia coli* – genes coding for the enzymes needed to utilize the sugar lactose – are normally inactive, but are switched on in the presence of lactose, enabling the bacterium to make use of this sugar. They found that there is a gene that codes for a 'regulatory protein' which, by virtue of its shape, can bind to the region of chromosome specifying the lactose enzymes, thereby switching off the necessary genes. Typically, therefore, the lactose enzymes are not produced. But, if there *is* lactose in the medium, lactose molecules bind to the regulatory protein, altering its shape, and thus preventing it from acting as a 'negative switch'. The result is that the enzyme-coding genes become active.

This discovery has become the model of how the activity of genes is regulated. In the particular case of the 'lac operon', regulation is negative, but we now know that regulation can also be positive: one gene can switch on another. One feature of such signalling systems, already clear to Monod, is that they are 'symbolic'.[8] By a 'symbol', semioticians mean a signal whose form is causally unrelated to its meaning. This is clear in the case of words. Thus in English the word 'cow' refers to a particular farm animal. But there is nothing in the sound of 'cow' that makes this meaning necessary – it could equally well mean a mountain or an article of clothing. A few words are not symbolic – 'cuckoo' for instance. But the meaning of most words is conventional. The same is true of genetic signals. The small-eye gene in the mouse means 'make an eye here', but, as far as its form is concerned, it could equally well mean 'make a whisker', or 'don't make a toe'.

Although Monod does not draw an explicit analogy between regulatory genes and the 'symbols' of the semioticians, the idea is implicit in his discussion. He points out that, although gene regulation necessarily depends on chemical reactions, there is no chemical necessity about which molecular signal induces which result. He calls this property 'gratuity', a term that is more apt in French than in English. It arises because a molecule that binds to one region on the surface of a protein can alter the overall shape of the protein. Hence natural selection can 'design' proteins that respond to the presence of a signal by altering their activity in any required way. This symbolic character of a signalling system is crucial, whether in the genetic code, in the control of development, or in human language. Only a symbolic system can convey an indefinitely large number of messages.

We now know that in higher organisms the activity of a particular gene may depend on the presence or absence of a number of proteins coded for by other genes. The idea of a network of regulatory genes is now well established. It is also an idea that fits well with Darwinism. Natural selection can alter body form by altering this network – by altering either a gene that codes for a regulatory signal, or the gene that receives the signal. But before describing how this works in more detail, I must discuss a second, very different idea, sometimes referred to as 'self-organization'.

CHAPTER 4

....

Information or Self-Organization?

Figure 1 shows a self-organized structure, formed when a small spherical object falls on the surface of a liquid. In what sense is it self-organized?

First, contrast it with the pattern shown in Figure 2.

This structure (at least in the form in which I sent it to the printer) was imposed on the paper by a stamp, which had the same structure (in fact, the business end of a potato-masher was painted, and then pressed on the paper). It is an example of 'template reproduction'. In template reproduction of biological structures, which are essentially three-dimensional, the 'positive' structure forms a negative, and the negative forms a new positive, but in each case the new structure is formed by contact

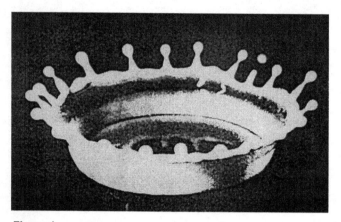

Figure 1
The splash pattern produced by dropping a small spherical object on the surface of a fluid.

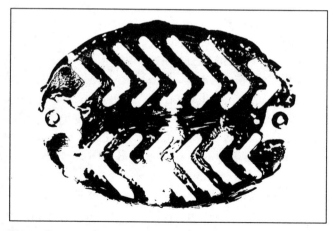

Figure 2
A pattern produced by 'template' reproduction.

22

with a pre-existing solid structure. One could say that a structure has been copied, but hardly that it has been generated. Such template reproduction is the basis of heredity: there is nothing 'self-organized' about it. But no one imagines that the structure of my hand, or eye, was formed in that way, any more than the bacterium *E. coli* was so formed.

But the idea of self-organization implies more than the simple fact that the structure was not punched out. Let us take another example. When my ink-jet printer prints a page of my manuscript, the structure on the page is in response to a stream of electrical impulses from my computer. To each dot on the paper there corresponded a particular electric impulse: change one impulse, and you would change one dot. In other words, the structure on the paper depended on the pre-existence of coded instructions. When geneticists say that development is genetically programmed, this is the idea they have in mind; when others say that it is self-organized, it is the idea that they are denying. The structure shown in Figure 1, then, is self-organized in two senses. It was not stamped out, and it did not require any specific instructions to make it. It is just the result of dynamical processes in the water, initiated by a falling drop. It could be said that the structure is too transient to be useful as an analogy for development: it is there for only a split second. But there are other self-organized structures that are long-lasting. I shall discuss one class of such structures, Turing waves, below.

There is, however, a more serious objection to the idea that biological structures are self-organized. Structures such as that illustrated in Figure 1 differ from biological structures in one crucial respect: they may be complicated, but they are not adapted to ensure their own survival and reproduction. It is this apparent design for survival that distinguishes living structures (and human artifacts) from non-living ones. An eye is designed for seeing: a vortex merely exists. This is a distinction that is ignored or underplayed by enthusiasts for self-organization. Biologists ignore Darwin at their peril. Certainly, processes analogous to those that gave rise to the splash pattern may occur in development; but if so, they will be pressed into the service of adaptive function. By altering genes, natural selection will alter the parameters – rates of reaction, diffusion, contraction and so on – so that a functional organ develops.

Perhaps the proponents of the genetic control of development are also leaving something out. Thus it is true that the form of the text on this page is adapted to convey my thoughts (I hope), and that it depended on a stream of coded instructions (in earlier days the text would have been stamped out, but that is so no longer). But it also depended on a complex machine, able to convert those instructions into patterns on paper. Genes cannot by themselves make an eye. What, then, is the analogue of the complex compositing machine? What do genes need before they can make an organism? Starting with a gene, we have a rather good understanding of how the sequence of bases in a gene is translated into the sequence of amino acids in a protein. It is true that this requires the existence of a complex structure, the ribosome (and some simpler structures), but since the molecules forming the ribosome are also coded for by genes, there is no great mystery here. (More precisely, there is no great mystery about the current maintenance and reproduction of the protein-synthesizing machinery: its evolutionary origin is a more difficult problem.) If all that was required for development was the synthesis of a large number of specific proteins, we could say that we understood development. There would, perhaps, be one caveat. Although we understand how genes specify the sequence of amino acids in a protein, there remains the problem of how the one-dimensional string of amino acids folds up to form a three-dimensional protein. In a sense, this is a problem not for biologists but for chemists. Most proteins will fold themselves up (although some require the assistance of accessory proteins, called chaperonins). In other words, the step from a one-dimensional string to a three-dimensional, functioning protein depends on the laws of physics, and an appropriate physical environment: it will happen in a test-tube. The genes do not have to code the laws of physics. Note, however, that we are invoking a dynamic process. It is one we would like to be able to simulate, because, for practical reasons, it would be extremely useful to be able to deduce the three-dimensional form of a protein from the base sequence of the gene coding for it; but this is still often beyond us. To summarize, we know in principle how the base sequence of a gene specifies the form of a protein, but a dynamical process of some complexity is involved.

The main difficulty, however, is that an organism is not merely a bag containing a number of different kinds of proteins. Even if its structure is, in the main, composed of proteins, they are arranged in a pattern in space. How does this pattern arise? It is not enough to say that different genes are switched on in different places, although this is true. We also need to know how the local action of specific genes is brought about. I will discuss this in a particular context: the early development of *Drosophila*.

In an early *Drosophila* embryo there are many nuclei, but cell walls have not yet appeared, and no structure is normally visible. The activity of a particular gene can be made visible by attaching fluorescent dyes to the RNA transcripts of these genes. In this way we can observe where two genes, *eve* (even-skipped) and *ftz* (fushi-tarazu), are active. The embryo has fourteen stripes in all, seven of *eve* and seven of *ftz* activity. Each of the stripes specifies the position of a segment in the adult. Later in development, they will each give rise to a segment, in total eight abdominal segments, three thoracic segments, and three anterior segments that will fuse to form the head region. (In fact, things are a bit more complicated, but the complications do not affect the present argument, so I will ignore them.) How does this pattern arise?

When I first observed this pattern of stripes in the *Drosophila* embryo, my immediate reaction was that I was looking at a wave with a series of peaks and troughs. Back in 1952, the mathematician Alan Turing (1912–54) had reached a rather counter-intuitive conclusion.[9] If a set of chemicals are present, and are able to react and to diffuse, one would expect the result to be a spatially uniform distribution of reactants: after all, diffusion leads to a net movement of molecules from regions of high to low concentration, and so to a uniform distribution. Indeed, this will usually be the case. Turing showed, however, that for some values of the reaction and diffusion rates, the uniform distribution is unstable, and a 'standing wave' of chemical concentrations will appear, with regularly spaced peaks and troughs of concentration. Quite recently, actual standing waves have been demonstrated in a test-tube. Turing referred to his chemicals as 'morphogens', and thought that they could be the basis of morphogenesis, perhaps responsible for the development of repeated structures such as the stripes of a zebra, insect segments or the petals of a flower. At the time, I was fascinated by Turing waves, and even interpreted (with rather weak supporting evidence) the arrangement of bristles on the cuticle of *Drosophila* as being responses to such waves.

It was therefore natural that I should have greeted the *Drosophila* embryo's stripes as confirmation of Turing's ideas. I was particularly delighted because I had predicted back in 1960 that, if the number of structures in different individuals were to be constant (we all have five fingers on each hand, and primroses have five petals per flower), the largest number that could be generated by a wave would be about seven.[10]

I think the argument in this paper is still of interest, even if insect segments are not induced by a Turing wave. I was interested in how the members of a species could always, or almost always, manage to generate the same fixed number of a repeated element – segments, vertebrae, fingers, petals. If the elements were induced by a wave, the number would be the nearest integer to the ratio (size of morphogenetic field) / (preferred wave length); the same point is made below in my discussion of the stripes on an angelfish. By looking at the accuracy with which continuous variables like height are regulated, I concluded that the largest number that could be generated repeatedly by this kind of 'ratio counting' was about seven. It is intriguing that the largest number of objects that an animal can learn to recognize is also about seven.

There are cases, however, in which animals successfully generate fixed numbers of repeated structures substantially larger than seven. The number of segments in insects and some other arthropods are examples. I suggested two ways in which this could be done. One was by 'multiplication': for example, first make seven segments, and then double each one. The other way I called 'qualitative counting': make each element qualitatively different from each other one. Given the vast quantity of information in the genome, this presents no difficulty in principle, although it involves a complicated signalling system. As will appear below, it seems that this is what flies do. The general point to emerge from all this is that only a rather small degree of morphological complexity (for example, seven similar structures, but not seventy) can be generated reliably in a single step; but, given enough genetic information, great complexity can be generated in a series of steps.

Thinking along these lines, I thought that, if an insect needed to generate fourteen segments, this would be too big a number to do in one step, but it could be done by multiplication: that is, by generating seven peaks, and using each peak to generate two structures. When, much later, I saw the embryo's stripes, it really seemed that *Drosophila* was doing what I had predicted.

Sadly, it seems that it is not so. If it was true, then each ring of activity of the gene *eve* would be induced by a peak of concentration of the same morphogen; but, as we shall see, this is not the case. Genetic analysis has revealed a much less elegant process.[11] If I got it wrong, it seems that Lewis Wolpert got it right.[12] He had suggested in 1969 (and earlier, in private conversation) a mechanism which, like Turing's, depended on diffusion. Suppose, he argued, you want to 'develop' the French flag – red, then white, then blue – on an initially uniform sheet of cells. First, set up a gradient of some chemical substance or morphogen: the easy way would be to produce it at one edge of the sheet, and allow it to diffuse, thus setting up a monotonic gradient. Then arrange that the gene responsible for the red pigment is switched on only by a high concentration of the morphogen, and that responsible for the blue pigment only at low concentrations: intermediate regions, with no pigment, would be white. More generally, his idea was that genes could be switched on or off by concentration gradients of morphogens, set up by diffusion.

It seems that, essentially, this is what is happening during the early development of *Drosophila*. The first antero-posterior gradient is set up by the *Bicoid* gene, which is active in the nurse cells that supply nutrients to the *Drosophila* egg as it grows in the ovary. When a gene is active, its base sequence is first copied, or 'transcribed', to a 'messenger RNA' molecule (mRNA), which passes out of the nucleus to the cell cytoplasm, where it is 'translated' into the amino acid sequence of a protein. The mRNA transcript of the gene is introduced into what is to be the anterior pole of the egg. There it is translated into Bicoid protein, which diffuses backwards through the egg, setting up a concentration gradient of precisely the kind imagined by Wolpert. After that, things get complicated. The details need not concern us. The essential point is that there is a cascade of gene activation and repression, first of the 'gap' genes (so-called because, when the function of one of these genes is destroyed by mutation, some structures fail to appear, leaving a gap in the usual antero-posterior array of structures), then of the 'pair rule' genes (*eve* and *ftz*), and then the Hox genes, which cause appropriate structures to develop on particular segments. Localized activation of genes occurs because each generation of genes is activated at particular positions in response to gradients set up by earlier genes in the cascade.

So how does the remarkable regularity of the pattern observed on the *Drosophila* embryo arise? It seems that the natural assumption − that *eve*, for example, is switched on by seven successive peaks of concentration of the same morphogen − is wrong. Instead, each ring of activation of *eve* occurs in response to a different combination of regulators; that is, each ring is differently regulated.

What are we to make of all this? If the pattern arose in response to a Turing wave, it would be a beautiful example of a rather complex pattern arising through a dynamic system. It would not be fully 'self-organized', because it would depend, among other things, on enzymes, which in turn are specified by genetic information. But it would be a nice illustration of the way in which genes can generate patterns by determining the parameters of dynamic systems (in this case, rates of reaction and diffusion). It now seems, however, that *Drosophila* segments are not specified in this way. Of course, they are not specified without the intervention of dynamics: after all, the diffusion of the Bicoid protein, and of other gene products, is a dynamic process. The difference is that, in the case of a wave, you get a more complex structure in a single step. But I cannot see that the difference between the two points of view is as profound as its protagonists sometimes appear to think.

Although it now seems that *Drosophila* segments are not specified by a Turing wave, it does not follow that such waves are never relevant. Clearly, it would be absurd to suppose that each segment, or pair of segments, in a centipede with over 150 segments is differently specified, as the segments of flies appear to be. But the segments of centipedes are not formed by subdividing an initially uniform field, as is the case in *Drosophila*: they are budded off sequentially at the anterior end. The process requires a temporal oscillation (just as the rhythmical movements of a skuller leave a series of dimples in the water behind him), but not a standing wave. One clue to the presence of a wave is provided when 'mistakes' are made. Take the example of a sea urchin bought by my wife and myself for sixpence on Penzance pier, in the days when I was obsessed by Turing waves. Although most echinoderms have had a 5-radial symmetry as adults since the Cambrian, and although that is the typical pattern for the sea urchin, this particular specimen has *six* perfect rays. The natural explanation is that, whether for genetic or environmental reasons we do not know, a wave with six peaks rather than five was formed, inducing six rays. If so, it would be senseless to ask which is the additional ray. But this explanation may be quite wrong.

A more convincing example of a Turing wave in a living system is afforded by the angelfish, *Pomacanthus*.[13] These fish have a rather regular array of stripes, vertical in *P. semicirculatus* and horizontal in *P. imperator*. The striking observation is that the number of stripes changes as the fish grows. Juvenile *P. semicirculatus* are less than 2 cm long, and have three vertical stripes. As the fish grows, the spacing between the stripes increases, until the fish is about 4 cm long. Then new stripes appear between the original ones, restoring the original spacing. The fish continues to grow and new stripes again appear between the existing ones when a length of about 8–9 cm is reached.

This differs from the situation in mammals, in which a skin colour pattern, once it appears, remains constant, merely increasing in size as the animal grows: an adult zebra has the same number of stripes as a juvenile. The appearance of new stripes in *Pomacanthus* can be expected if the mechanism underlying the pattern is the one suggested by Turing, and if the chemical reactions generating the wave continue throughout life. The reason is as follows. Given the reaction and diffusion rates, there is a 'preferred' spacing between stripes. The actual number formed will depend on the size of the region in which reaction and diffusion can occur. As the size of the region increases, so does the expected number of wave peaks. Thus the pattern changes observed during growth are predicted by the Turing mechanism. The snag is that they would be predicted equally well by any other process that could generate a wave – for example, waves can be generated by mechanical forces or by cell movements. The importance of the angelfish example is that, if it is a Turing wave, it should be possible to identify the morphogens. Biologists are not going to believe it until this happens.

Perhaps the clearest evidence that complex patterns can appear as the result of dynamic processes, without the need for localized gene action, comes from the study of organisms with only a single nucleus: in such organisms, there may be variation in gene activity in time, but not in space. I will illustrate the complexity that can arise in such single-celled organisms by the example of the marine alga, *Acetabularia*, because I am familiar with the research, some of which was carried out by Brian Goodwin, in collaboration with Lynn Trainor, when he was my colleague at Sussex.[14]

Acetabularia acetabulum is a marine alga which grows from a single cell anchored to the substrate by a branching rootlet, which houses the single nucleus in one of its branches. From this base there grows a single slender stalk. When this stalk has reached 1–1.5 cm, a ring of buds is formed which develops into a whorls of branched leaflets. The stalk continues to grow from the centre of the whorl and new whorls of leaflets are produced at irregular intervals. Finally a sculptured cap – the 'mermaid's cap' of the common name – is formed at the tip, and the leaflets are shed, giving an adult some 3–5 cm high.

Clearly, this structure cannot depend on different

genes being active at different places: there is only one nucleus. Gene products are carried up the stem by cytoplasmic streaming. So what is going on? We do not have a complete answer: in particular, the formation of the cap remains a mystery. But Goodwin and Trainor did come up with a model which can explain the lateral leaflets. The model incorporates some essential features of the growing stalk. The centre of the stalk is occupied by a fluid-filled vacuole. The cytoplasm is confined to a thin outer layer, bounded by an inner and outer membrane, and surrounded by a cell wall. The crucial point is that the cytoplasm contains both elastic and contractile protein fibres. Its stiffness and contractility depend in a non-linear fashion on calcium concentration. There is also a feedback system, because contraction of the cytoplasm alters calcium concentration. In other words, the stalk is a hollow fluid-filled tube with a wall which is elastic, but whose elasticity is altered by its own contraction and relaxation. Goodwin and Trainor computer-simulated the results of such a system, allowing for the way in which the elasticity and contractility of the outer cytoplasm is influenced by calcium concentration, and itself reacts back on the calcium concentration. As the symmetrical dome grows, the calcium concentration, initially at a maximum in the centre, forms a ring of high concentration.

After a period of growth, the tip flattens out. If, at this stage, a slight perturbation of the calcium concentration is made, this leads to the appearance of a ring of peaks of concentration. If a comparable ring of peaks arose in a living alga, they would give rise to a ring of leaflike lateral outgrowths.

The formal similarity between the growth of *Acetabularia* and the ring of droplets shown in Figure 1 is not an accident. I chose Figure 1 deliberately. The details of the dynamic systems giving rise to the two patterns are, of course, quite different, but two points do emerge. First, rather simple rules can give rise to relatively complex patterns. Second, similar patterns can arise from different sets of rules.

I do not think it is sensible to speak of the growth of *Acetabularia* as self-organized. Of course it is self-organized in the sense that no-one else is organizing it. But as I explained earlier, the term carries with it the notion that there is no information or set of instructions specifying the structure. But in this case growth depends on the presence of many specific proteins – for example, those responsible for cell wall growth, elasticity and contractility. These proteins require genetic information. Changes in genes can alter the parameters of the system (for example, the elastic modulus of the cytoplasm), and by so doing can alter the morphology. So, unlike the splash pattern, the form of *Acetabularia* depends on coded information.

But a pattern can depend on information in many different ways. I want to consider three examples: the pattern of letters on this page; the form of *Acetabularia*; and the segments of *Drosophila*.

First, consider the letters on this page. It would be

possible to point to the specific signal responsible for the following letter, A. Change that particular signal, and you would change the A, and nothing else. Some biological information is like that. Change a particular base in the DNA, and you will change a particular amino acid in a particular protein. However, that amino acid change may have manifold effects later in development. Thus there is a one-to-one correspondence between a triplet of bases in the DNA and an amino acid, but not between amino acid and a particular feature of adult morphology. I think that when Goodwin, for example, objects to the notion of the genetic programming of development, it is this one-to-one correspondence that he objects to.

Next, consider morphogenesis in *Acetabularia*. Certainly, one cannot point to particular genes that are responsible for particular morphological features. Instead, genes set the parameters of a dynamic system, which then generates the form.

In the development of *Drosophila*, and multicellular organisms generally, the way in which genetic information is made use of differs from that in single-celled organisms like *Tetrahymena* and *Acetabularia* in two important ways. First, although (with a few exceptions) all cells contain a complete set of genes, different genes are active in different cells. Even a structure such as the fourteen stripes of the *Drosophila* embryo, which looks as if it is the outcome of a single dynamic process, in fact depends on the successive activation of different sets of genes in different places, a possibility not open to *Acetabularia*.

Multicellularity offers a second information-translating device which I have not yet mentioned explicitly. Once a set of genes has been switched on or off in a cell, this state of activation can be transmitted to daughter cells arising by division of the original cell. Such cells are said to be 'differentiated'. We are beginning to understand the way in which states of activation are transmitted. Chemical 'labels' are attached to genes, altering their activity, and these labels are copied when the cell divides and the genes are replicated. But what matters here is the result, not the mechanism. The result is that development can be divided into a series of successive processes of differentiation. Each process of differentiation starts with a set of similar cells, and ends with two or more sets of cells with different potentialities and different ultimate fates. This has an important consequence. The amount of morphological complexity that can be added in a single developmental step is relatively small if 'mistakes' are to be avoided: the mistake that was made by the sea urchin mentioned earlier shows that things can go wrong if too much complexity is added in one go. The complex morphology of an adult *Drosophila* does not arise out of a single dynamical process affecting the whole organism, but in a series of steps, with the later steps affecting only small parts of the organism, and utilizing genetic information specific to that part.

In other words, during development the embryo is successively divided into smaller and smaller regions, whose subsequent growth is to a degree autonomous, although signals do pass between regions, serving to integrate the whole process. This modularity of development, which I discussed earlier, is imposed on complex organisms by the need for accuracy and repeatability. As I pointed out then, however, modularity has important consequences for evolution. On the one hand, it makes it possible for one part to change without altering every part, thus making gradual evolution possible. On the other, it helps to explain the conservation of the body plans of the different phyla, represented by their 'phylotypic stages'.

Does this mean that those interested in the development of multicellular animals and plants can forget about the kind of pattern formation postulated for *Acetabularia* and other single-celled organisms? I do not think so. I have already argued that even a well-understood process such as protein synthesis involves a little-understood dynamic process of folding. The simple 'French flag' model explains much of early development in *Drosophila*, but it also requires the dynamic process of diffusion. The difference is that diffusion, although a dynamic process, is a very boring one, hardly worthy of the name, whereas the processes responsible for the pattern in Figure 1 and the growth of *Acetabularia acetabulum* are exciting, generating unexpected results. It would not be safe to assume that interesting dynamic processes do not occur in higher organisms. On the other hand, those interested in dynamic systems and self-organization cannot afford to ignore the 10^9 bits of information stored in the genome – the quantity of information contained in several hundred books.

CHAPTER 5

....

Reductionists to the Right, Holists to the Left

I have described two approaches to the study of development. One is global, holistic and dynamic; the other is local, reductionist, and dependent on notions of information, regulation and control. Such a division is not peculiar to developmental biology. I recently attended a workshop jointly organized by neurobiologists and computer scientists on how brains, natural and artificial, may work, and was intrigued to find a similar debate between a 'program-oriented' and a 'dynamic systems' school. The former see a necessary parallel between the way the brain works and the way a computer program is written. Adaptive behaviour by an animal, or a robot, requires that it have knowledge of the world – for example, navigation in space requires that there be a 'cognitive map' in its head. Particular concepts must be represented by specific structures in the program, and there must be a flow of logic of the form 'If X is true, do A; if not, do B'. The latter, dynamic systems school are more impressed by the fact that, in a computer, neural nets 'learn' to solve problems in ways that are not obvious to the programmer, and in which it is hard to identify particular connections in the net with particular decisions. Adaptive behaviour, they argue, does not require knowledge of the world, but only a set of appropriate reactions to immediate stimuli. Such debates are perhaps inevitable, so long as it is true that both approaches are possible and occasionally fruitful, and so long as most of us find it hard to think simultaneously in two such different ways. I want to end by describing a curious, but apparently unavoidable, ideological component to such debates.

Let me start with a personal anecdote. In 1950 at University College London, I attended lectures on genetics by Hans Gruneberg (1907–83). He was a convinced, and convincing, proponent of the view that 'genes control development'. One day I put on the notice board in the student laboratory a cartoon of horses pulling a carriage, driven by Gruneberg (who was rather easy to caricature) wielding a whip, with the caption 'genes control development'. The point of this story is that I was in those days a Marxist, albeit one whose faith was rapidly crumbling. I disliked the idea of one-way control, and preferred a more cooperative and interactive picture of development. As I have become more critical of Marxism, so I have become more of a reductionist in science. I do not assert that there is a causal connection, but I suspect there may be: if there is, I don't know which way the causation goes. Certainly, those of my friends who favour a holistic approach also tend to be politically on the left. I'm not sure the generalization holds in North America, and I certainly do not claim that all my reductionist friends are right-wing. But I am fairly confident that there is an association between holistic views about development and left-wing political opinions. The association is not just with left-wing opinions. Recently, reading Evelyn Fox-Keller's *Secrets of Life, Secrets of Death*, I was fascinated to find a feminist critic of science equating the reductionist approach of molecular biology with the aim of male domination of 'nature', where 'nature' was thought to be female.[15]

The immediate reaction of most scientists to such imputations of ideological bias will be that, in so far as it exists, it should be resisted. Scientific issues should be decided by the evidence, not by ideological bias. Of course I agree, but I also suspect that the matter is not quite as simple as it looks. If two people as intelligent and well-informed as embryologists Brian Goodwin and Lewis Wolpert can disagree so profoundly, the issue between them cannot be settled all that easily. Part of the difficulty is that the debate is not so much an argument about what the world is like, as about the best way to pursue one's research. So long as there is more than one potentially fruitful approach to a problem, there will be disagreements. It is easy for me, as an outsider who is not going to devote time and energy to experiments in this field, to say that an understanding of development is going to require both a dynamical and an informational approach: it is much harder for someone who is going to do some real work.

This book is based on a lecture given at the London School of Economics. I must end, therefore, by pointing to a curious paradox. In developmental biology, to believe in self-organization seems to be associated with left-wing or feminist views. Not so in economics. Surely the perfect example of a theory asserting that a well-adapted structure emerges not from central planning and control but from the free self-interested behaviour of individuals, is the notion of the 'hidden hand' propounded by the Scottish economist Adam Smith (1723–90). If individuals are free to buy and sell what they want, to work for whom they wish, and to invest where they will, the result will be an economic system in which the goods that people want are efficiently produced. I am not competent to discuss the validity of this theory, although I am tempted to point out that it may be profitable to pour poison into rivers, to advertize cigarettes and to sell alcoholic drinks to small children. My point is that an association between theories of self-organization on the one hand and political orientation on the other, which appears to exist in biology, is reversed in economics.

For biologists, I think that the moral is that it pays to be eclectic in our choice of theories. Of course, we have to avoid believing simultaneously in two contradictory theories, or in any one theory that is contradicted by observations that we think are correct. But this leaves plenty of room to be reductionist in one context and holist in another. Inevitably, and with reason, scientists are influenced by success. I remarked earlier that I have tended to become more reductionist as I have grown older. This may have something to do with a progressive disenchantment with Marxism, but I think the main reason is the obvious success of molecular biology in explaining evolution and embryology. But I think it is valuable for scientists to have a well-furnished mind. It is important for biologists to know some physics, not just because some piece of physics may be relevant to the problem they are working on, but because physics is the best exemplar we have of the kinds of theories that can exist, and of the ways they may explain reality. But it is also important for physical scientists moving into biology to be aware that they are entering a strange territory, in which two unfamiliar concepts – adaptation and information – are central.

NOTES
....

1 Maynard Smith, J., *The Problems of Biology* (Oxford University Press, 1986).

2 Halder, G., Callaerts, P. and Gehring, W. J., 'Induction of ectopic eyes by targeted expression of the *eyeless* gene in *Drosophila*' (*Science*, 267: 1788–92, 1995). For a discussion of what the experiment tells us about evolution, see Nilsson, D-E. (*Current Biology* 6: 39–42, 1996).

3 Slack, J. M. W., Holland, P. W. H. and Graham, C. F., 'The zootype and the phylotypic stage' (*Nature* 361: 490–2, 1993).

4 Appel, T. A., *The Cuvier-Geoffroy Debate* (Oxford University Press, 1987). This book starts with the following anecdote, which illustrates the philosophical importance then held by morphology. Shortly after the Revolution of 1830 had removed Charles X from the French throne, Frederic Soret visited his friend Goethe. 'Now', Goethe exclaimed, 'what do you think of this great event? The volcano has come to eruption; everything is in flames, and we no

longer have a transaction behind closed doors!' To his astonishment, Soret found that Goethe was speaking, not of the July Revolution, but of the opening of the debate between Cuvier and Geoffroy.

5 Holley, S. A. *et al.* (*Nature* 376: 249–53, 1995).

6 Raff, R. A., *The Shape of Life: Genes, Development and the Evolution of Animal Form* (University of Chicago Press, 1996). Contains an excellent discussion of the conservation of the phylotypic stage, despite changes earlier, and later, in development. Raff's own work on echinoderms shows how early development can evolve rapidly, from a life history involving a small egg and a planktonic larval stage to one with a large yolky egg and direct development, while preserving a relatively unchanged adult form.

7 Jacob, F. & Monod, J., 'On the regulation of gene activity' (*Cold Spring Harbour Symposia on Quantitative Biology* 26: 193–211, 1961).

8 Jacques Monod's *Chance and Necessity*, first published in France in 1970 and recently reissued in English translation by Penguin Books.

9 Turing, A. M., 'The chemical basis of morphogenesis' (*Phil. Trans. Roy. Soc.* B237: 37–72, 1952). An intuitive explanation of Turing's idea, explaining the circumstances in which a wave will appear, is given in Maynard Smith, J., *Mathematical Ideas in Biology* (Cambridge University Press, 1968, pp. 123–5).

10 Maynard Smith, J., 'Continuous, quantized and

modal variation' (*Proc. Roy. Soc.* B152: 397–409, 1960).

11 Akam, M., 'Making stripes inelegantly' (*Nature* 341: 282–3, 1989). An elegant account of this problem.

12 Wolpert, L., 'Positional information and the pattern of cellular differentiation' (*J. Theor. Biol.* 25: 1–47, 1969).

13 Kondo, S. and Rihito, A., 'A reaction-diffusion wave on the skin of the marine angelfish *Pomacanthus*' (*Nature* 376: 765–8, 1995).

14 Webster, G. and Goodwin, B., *Form and Transformation: Generative and Relational Principles in Biology* (Cambridge University Press, 1996).

15 Fox Keller, E., *Secrets of Life, Secrets of Death* (Routledge, NY: 1992). It is interesting that Fox Keller's own earlier work in biology had been on the aggregation of individual cells of the slime mould, *Dictyostelium*, to form a migrating 'slug'. This is one of the cases in biology in which a holistic model has proved illuminating.

SUGGESTIONS FOR FURTHER READING

Appel, T. A., *The Cuvier-Geoffroy Debate* (Oxford University Press, 1987).

Fox Keller, E., *Secrets of Life, Secrets of Death* (Routledge, NY: 1992).

Lawrence, P. A., *The Making Of A Fly* (Blackwell Science, 1992). A fascinating if rather technical account of *Drosophila* development.

Maynard Smith, J., *Mathematical Ideas in Biology* (Cambridge University Press, 1968).

Maynard Smith, J., *The Problems of Biology* (Oxford University Press, 1986).

Monod, Jacques, *Chance and Necessity* (Penguin, 1997).

Raff, R. A., *The Shape of Life: Genes, Development and the Evolution of Animal Form* (University of Chicago Press, 1996).

Thompson, D'Arcy, *On Growth and Form* (Cambridge University Press, 1917).

Webster, G. and Goodwin, B., *Form and Transformation: Generative and Relational Principles in Biology* (Cambridge University Press, 1996).

Wolpert, L., *The Triumph of the Embryo* (Oxford University Press, 1991). A good, non-technical introduction.